"Beyond Labels: A Parent's Guide to Gender Diversity"

"A Comprehensive Resource for Families, Schools, and Children on Understanding and Addressing Gender and Sexual Identity"

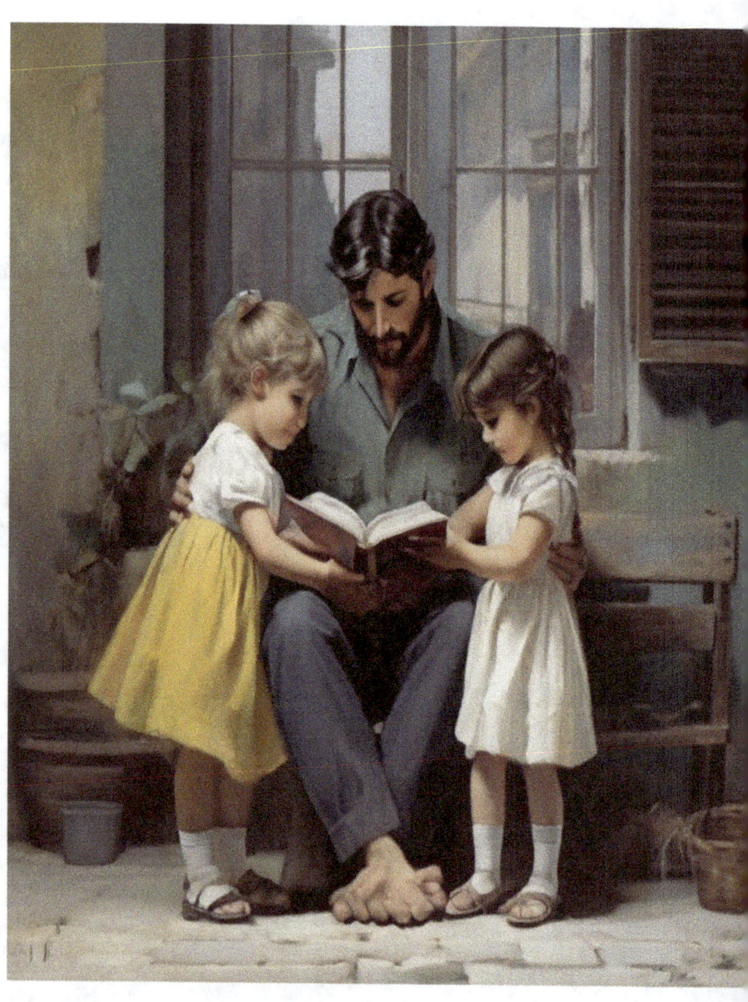

Table of Contents: "Beyond Labels: A Parent's Guide to Gender Diversity"

- Educational Resources to Facilitate Dialogue

- In-depth Insights: Practical Advice from Psychologists

4.Recognizing and Supporting Gender Diversity in Children

- Identifying Precious Signs

- Supporting Exploration of Gender Identity

- Managing Family Dynamics

- Practical Tools: Creating an Accepting Environment

5. Daily Actions to Foster a Welcoming Environment

- Empathetic and Respectful Language

- Creating Spaces for Individual Expression

- Modifying the Dynamics of Games and Activities

- Open Dialogues on Positive Role Models

8. Explaining Gender Diversity to Children with Sensitivity

- Creating an Open Space for Conversation

- Using Age-Appropriate Language

- Promoting Acceptance and Kindness

- Introducing Positive Stories

- Responding to Specific Questions

Final Chapter: Beyond Labels, Toward a Future of Acceptance

- Final Reflections: The Uniqueness of Each Individual

- The Power of Unconditional Acceptance

- Looking Ahead: Building an Inclusive Future

- Heartfelt Thanks

- Additional Resources: Continuing the Journey

- Conclusion: A Never-ending Journey

Bonus Additional Chapter: Exploring One's Gender and Sexual Identity

For Adults:

Self-Awareness and Reflection:

- How to Begin Exploring One's Gender and Sexual Identity

- Personal Reflections and Self-awareness

Psychological Resources:

- Advice from Psychologists Specialized in Gender and Sexual Identity

- Professional Support for Addressing Doubts and Uncertainties

2Community and Support Groups:

- Engaging in Online Communities or Local Support Groups

- Sharing Experiences and Connecting with Individuals who have faced similar situations

For Children:

Open and Welcoming Dialogues:

- Creating an Open Family Environment to Discuss Gender and Sexual Identity

- The Importance of Non-Judgmental Dialogue

School Inclusion:

- How Schools Can Promote an Inclusive and Welcoming Environment

- Tips for Educators and Teachers on Addressing Children's Questions and Concerns

Parental Involvement:

- Active Parental Involvement in Supporting Children's Exploration of their Identity

- Practical Resources and Tips for Parents

Practical Advice for Everyone:

Reading and Educational Resources:

- Books and Educational Resources Suitable for All Ages to Better Understand Gender and Sexual Identity

- Tips on Effectively Using Such Resources

Responsible Online Research:

Introduction:

Welcome to our guide, "Beyond Labels: A Parent's Guide to Gender Identity." Gender identity is an important aspect of human diversity, and understanding this concept is crucial for building an inclusive and respectful society. This booklet has been created with the aim of providing parents with the necessary tools to explain the transgender reality to their children in an educational and compassionate manner. The world is evolving, and with it, our perceptions of gender are also changing. Through this guide, we hope to provide clear information and practical advice to help families navigate gender identity conversations openly, warmly, and lovingly. We are confident that, with understanding and support, we can build a future where every individual feels free to be themselves, without fear or prejudice.

Chapter 1: What Is Gender Identity?

Gender identity is a fundamental concept for understanding human diversity. When we talk about gender identity, we refer to how a person internally identifies in terms of male, female, or other gender identities. It is crucial to distinguish between gender identity and biological sex, as the latter refers to physical characteristics such as genital organs, chromosomes, and hormones.

Imagine gender identity as the way a person feels they belong to the world, recognizing themselves internally. Some people identify with the gender assigned to them at birth (male or female), while others may experience a different gender identity. It is important to understand that gender identity is not limited to the male/female binary; there are many diverse gender identities, including non-binary, bigender, agender, and many others.

In summary, gender identity is a deep and personal aspect of who we are. Respect for this diversity contributes to creating an environment where each individual feels acknowledged and accepted for their unique identity. In the next section, we will explore the concept of transgender and how it relates to gender identity.

Chapter 2: The Difference between Sex and Gender

Introduction:

In our journey to fully understand gender diversity, it is crucial to lay the groundwork with a clear distinction between two often-confused concepts: sex and gender. While sex refers to the biological and physical characteristics that distinguish individuals as male or female, gender is a social construct that goes beyond these anatomical distinctions, involving how individuals identify and express themselves.

Sex: Beyond Biology

Sex, often identified at birth based on physical criteria such as genital organs and chromosomes, is an aspect of our identity that can have a range of nuances. It is important to recognize that biological sex does not always uniquely determine an individual's gender. For example, some individuals may be born with physical characteristics that do not align with their internal sense of being male or female.

Gender: The Social Construct

Gender, on the other hand, is based on cultural, social, and behavioral expectations associated with males and females. It is a complex concept that encompasses gender identity, gender expression, and gender roles. While sex is assigned at birth, gender is an individual construct that can evolve throughout a person's life.

In-depth Exploration: Cultural Differences in Gender Identity

Conceptions of gender can vary significantly across different cultures. Some societies may recognize more than two gender categories, while others may have strict expectations tied to male and female roles. Exploring these differences can enrich our understanding of gender diversity.

The Evolution of Understanding

Our understanding of sex and gender is continually evolving. Modern society is increasingly recognizing the diversity of gender identities, pushing us to challenge traditional norms. With scientific and social progress, we are paving the way for a more inclusive and respectful view of gender diversity.

Who Are Transgender People?

The concept of transgender is a fundamental element in understanding gender identity. Transgender individuals are those who experience a disconnect between the 2gender identity they identify with and the sex assigned to them at birth. In other words, a transgender person may be born with a body that does not reflect their internal gender identity.

The Challenge of Misunderstanding:

Many transgender people face unique challenges in trying to make others understand their experience. Often, society may be limited by rigid gender norms, making it difficult for transgender individuals to be recognized and respected in their identity.

The Variance of Transgender Experience:

It is crucial to note that the transgender experience is highly individual. Each transgender person has their own story, perception, and way of dealing with their gender identity. Some individuals may undergo physical transition through hormone use or surgeries, while others may choose to express their gender identity through clothing and behaviors.

Acceptance and Support:

Transgender individuals, especially during processes of self-acceptance and sharing with others, seek an environment of acceptance and support. The role of parents becomes crucial in this context, as family support can make a difference in the emotional and mental well-being of a transgender individual.

Positive Experience Narratives:

Introducing stories of success and acceptance can be a powerful way to debunk myths and break down prejudices. This chapter includes narratives of positive transgender experiences, highlighting the courage and resilience of those who have embraced their gender identity.

Story 1: The Courage to Embrace Your Child's Gender Identity

Maria and Paolo, a couple of parents who strongly believed in the importance of creativity and open-mindedness, were taken by surprise when Marco revealed his desire to explore gender identity. Initially confused and worried, Maria and Paolo decided to embark on a journey of understanding. They began with specialized psychological counseling, attending sessions together to learn how to support Marco.

The key moment arrived when Marco, with the courage that only young people can have, organized a "heart-to-heart" evening with his parents. He shared his feelings, experiences, and challenges faced in discovering his identity. Marco used his artistic talent to visually illustrate his feelings, opening a dialogue that helped build a bridge between him and his parents. Over time, through open conversations and continuous support, Marco's family demonstrated that unconditional love and acceptance are the cornerstones of their bond.

Story 2: Acceptance and Growth through Unconditional Love

Giulia and Luca, a couple of parents passionate about artistic expression, experienced an emotional storm when Alice, their intelligent and passionate daughter, revealed being transgender. Initially confused, Giulia and Luca rushed to seek help from a specialized psychologist. Alice found the courage to organize a family evening where she shared her experiences, fears, and hopes for the future. She presented a song, written to express her identity, touching the hearts of her parents and opening a window into her soul. Giulia and Luca decided to support Alice with unconditional love, turning this journey into an opportunity for growth and learning for the entire family.

Story 3: A Journey of Self-Discovery for the Whole Family

Matteo, a young artist from a family passionate about creative exploration, shared his gender identity with Sofia and Roberto, parents who value diversity and freedom of expression. The beginning of the journey was marked by a family evening where Matteo showcased his artworks, each representing a chapter of his self-discovery journey. The family embarked on a collective reading of educational books on gender diversity and participated in workshops that fueled mutual understanding. Matteo had the courage to initiate dialogue, showing Sofia and Roberto that open communication and acceptance can transform challenges into opportunities for family growth and connection.

In this chapter, we laid the foundations for a deeper understanding of gender diversity, clearly outlining the differences between sex and gender. We now continue our journey, exploring how loving parents can navigate through this complex and fascinating dimension of their children's lives.

Continuing to explore the transgender world, we help families understand that, through respect and awareness, we can contribute to creating a more inclusive and welcoming environment for everyone. In the next chapter, we will discuss how parents can address and explain the transgender reality to their sons.

Chapter 3: Open Conversations and Family Acceptance

Introduction:

We are now entering a crucial chapter of our journey: how to initiate and maintain open conversations about gender diversity with our children. Family understanding and acceptance are fundamental cornerstones to support children in their unique paths of exploring gender identity.

Initial Conversations: Creating a Welcoming Environment

The start of this conversation might be a sensitive moment, yet it is essential. Loving parents can create a safe and welcoming environment, letting their children know that they are ready to listen without judgment. Affectionately embracing children's revelations is crucial to building trust and connection.

Insights: Practical Tips from Psychologists

Experienced psychologists suggest staying calm and expressing support. Avoiding overly emotional reactions can promote a more open and comfortable dialogue.

Navigating Emotions: For Parents and Children

Gender diversity can evoke a range of emotions in both parents and children. Feeling confused, worried, or even scared is normal. Openly sharing these emotions can strengthen the family bond and demonstrate authentic commitment to acceptance.

Deepening Understanding: Shared Readings and Educational Resources

To facilitate dialogue, we might integrate shared readings and educational resources on gender diversity. Books and materials suitable for children's ages can be helpful in explaining complex concepts in an accessible way.

Building a Lasting Connection

The chapter concludes by emphasizing the importance of building a lasting connection. Gender diversity is an evolving journey, and continuous support and unconditional love from parents are crucial for the emotional well-being of their children.

How to Explain to Children?

Addressing the topic of gender diversity with children requires delicacy and clarity. To guide this process, it is helpful to draw on expert advice and use concrete examples to make the topic more understandable.

Simplify Without Reducing:

Children have a surprising capacity to understand complex concepts, but it is essential to adapt the language to their comprehension abilities. An example could be explaining that "some children feel more comfortable dressing differently from what others expect, and that's okay."

Stories and Analogies:

Narratives are powerful educational tools. Use stories involving transgender characters positively, emphasizing acceptance and love. For example, you could tell the story of a character discovering their gender identity and receiving support from family and friends.

Answering Questions:

Children will likely have many questions. Psychologists advise answering honestly and age-appropriately, tailoring responses to the child's level of understanding. For instance, you could respond to a question about gender diversity by saying, "Just like there are many types of flowers in the garden, there are also many types of people, and each one is special in their own way."

Normalizing Diversity:

Respect and normalize gender diversity. Psychologists recommend using positive examples in everyday life, such as the various activities children can engage in regardless of gender. For example, you could emphasize that children can love playing with dolls or toy cars, regardless of gender.

Demonstrate Respect:

Psychologists emphasize the crucial role of parents in modeling respect. Through respectful behaviors and language, children learn to be open and tolerant. For instance, you could positively comment on gender diversity in media or in your daily interactions.

By incorporating advice from psychologists and using concrete examples, parents can create an environment where children learn the importance of respect and understanding for all gender identities. In the next chapter, we will explore the crucial role of parents in supporting and accepting their transgender children more deeply.

In this chapter, we have explored how to initiate and maintain open conversations about gender diversity, providing practical tips from psychologists and educational resources. Let's now continue our journey, delving more deeply into the practical and psychological dynamics of this path.

Chapter 4: Recognizing and Supporting Gender Diversity in Children

Introduction:

We now delve into more practical territory, exploring how loving parents can identify and support gender diversity in their children. This chapter provides a detailed analysis of signals, family dynamics, and practical tools to navigate this journey of understanding and acceptance.

Recognizing Precious Signals

1.1 From toy choices to clothing preferences: Parents can learn to recognize valuable signals that provide precious insights into the child's internal perception.

1.2 Insights from Psychologists: Psychologists advise paying attention to the consistency of signals and avoiding rigid gender stereotypes. An open and non-judgmental approach is crucial to fully understand the child's experience.

Supporting Gender Identity Exploration

Loving parents can practically and empathetically support their children's exploration of gender identity. This may involve accessing educational resources, participating in support groups, and engaging in activities that encourage individual expression.

Family Dynamics: Open Dialogues and Acceptance

Open dialogue within the family is crucial. This chapter explores how parents can manage family dynamics by involving other members in a respectful and informative conversation about gender diversity.

Practical Tools: Creating an Accepting Environment

The chapter concludes by offering practical tools to create an accepting, inclusive, and respectful gender-diverse environment. From changes in family communication to small daily actions, these tools are designed to integrate acceptance into every aspect of family life.

The Role of Parents: Acceptance and Support

The role of parents in supporting transgender children is fundamental to fostering an environment of acceptance and understanding. Psychologists provide practical advice to help parents navigate this path.

Embracing the Child's Identity:

Embracing the child's gender identity means recognizing and respecting their self-identification. Experts emphasize that openly expressing support, such as saying "I love you for who you are" or "I'm here to support you," contributes to creating a positive bond between parent and child.

Creating a Supportive Environment:

Creating a supportive environment means not only accepting but also adapting to the child's needs and expressions. For example, if the child wishes to dress differently, providing clothing options and showing enthusiasm for their choices strengthens their sense of identity.

Being an Active Ally:

Being an active ally requires a constant commitment to education and support. Parents can attend seminars, read books on gender diversity, and actively engage in advocacy initiatives.

Open and Honest Communication:

Open communication is crucial. Psychologists recommend creating a safe space where the child feels free to express their experiences, emotions, and questions.

Tangible Examples of Support:

Demonstrating support in tangible ways helps the child feel understood and loved. Examples range from attending school events advocating gender diversity to providing informative resources.

Observing the Child:

Psychologists advise closely observing the child to identify signs of well-being or discomfort. A supportive environment should reflect in the child's behavior and mood.

Incorporating specific and practical examples helps parents better understand how to translate theoretical support into daily actions, thereby promoting an environment that fully welcomes and supports transgender children. In the next chapter, we will explore how to create an inclusive environment in both family and society.

In this chapter, we've explored how loving parents can recognize and support gender diversity in their children, providing practical advice from psychologists and educational resources. Let's continue our journey, examining further how understanding and acceptance can translate into daily actions.

Chapter 5: Empathetic and Respectful Language

Introduction:

Language holds immense power. In this chapter, we explore how empathetic and respectful language can contribute to creating an inclusive family environment. Avoiding gender stereotypes in daily conversations and encouraging an open and diverse vocabulary are foundational steps.

Insights: Advice from Psychologists

Active Listening and Sensitivity: Psychologists emphasize the importance of actively listening to children and responding sensitively to their linguistic needs. This practice can foster trust and open communication.

Creating Spaces for Individual Expression

Every child has the right to express their identity uniquely. We explore how loving parents can create spaces where their children feel free to express their individuality through clothing, room decoration, and creative activities.

Transforming the Dynamics of Games and Activities

In a world often characterized by gender stereotypes in games and activities, this chapter provides suggestions on how parents can modify dynamics to encourage a more open and inclusive experience.

Open Dialogues on Positive Role Models

Parents play a crucial role in presenting positive role models. This chapter examines how loving parents can engage in open dialogues about positive role models, encouraging equality and diversity.

Creating Inclusive Family Traditions

 Lastly, we explore how parents can create inclusive family traditions that celebrate gender diversity. From holidays to special occasions, these traditions can become pillars of acceptance and love.

Creating an Inclusive Environment

Creating an inclusive family environment is a crucial step in supporting transgender children and promoting a sense of acceptance and belonging. In this chapter, we will explore various strategies and practices that parents can adopt to create an inclusive and gender-diverse environment.

Continuous Education:

Experts highlight the importance of ongoing education for parents. Staying informed about gender diversity topics, following new research, and participating in workshops or conferences contribute to a deeper understanding.

Example: Reading books on gender diversity, attending informative webinars, and engaging in discussions with other parents can be effective ways to maintain continuous education.

Respectful Language:

The use of respectful and inclusive language is fundamental. Psychologists recommend avoiding gender stereotypes in language and using appropriate pronouns.

Example: Using correct pronouns when referring to the child and encouraging others to do the same contributes to creating a respectful environment.

Promoting Diversity in Toys and Media:

Introducing a variety of toys and educational materials that reflect gender diversity is a tangible way to promote inclusivity.

Example: Purchasing books and toys featuring characters of diverse gender identities and cultural backgrounds helps normalize diversity.

Valuing Differences:

Experts advise promoting a family culture that values individual differences and celebrates diversity as enrichment.

Example: Encouraging the child to explore their interests, regardless of traditional gender roles, demonstrates acceptance of their individual choices.

Community Engagement:

Being an active part of communities that promote inclusivity can have a significant impact. Psychologists suggest participating in events, support groups, and advocacy initiatives.

Example: Joining parent groups supporting gender diversity can offer mutual support and contribute to creating a network of solidarity.

Addressing Bullying and Prejudice:

Experts recommend preparing the child to face bullying and prejudice that may arise. Creating an environment where the child feels supported and understood helps develop resilience.

Example: Open discussion and preparation for handling challenging situations can prepare the child to navigate potential difficulties.

In this chapter, we've explored the daily actions that loving parents can take to create an authentically welcoming and respectful family environment for gender diversity. Let's now continue our journey, heading toward a deeper and more practical understanding of how to apply these principles in everyday life.

Chapter 6: Deep Connections and Sustainability

Introduction:

In our journey towards a practical and profound understanding of gender diversity, we delve further into family connections and the importance of sustainability in the environment we've created. This chapter explores the psychological and practical dimensions of maintaining deep and sustainable connections.

Understanding Evolving Emotions

Emotions can evolve over time, for both parents and children. In this chapter, we delve into how loving parents can understand and manage evolving emotions, creating a safe space for emotional growth.

Insights: Psychologists' Advice

Psychologists emphasize the importance of adapting to the changing emotional needs of children, providing consistent support, and encouraging open communication.

Supporting Individual Growth

Individual growth is an integral part of gender diversity. Loving parents can support the individual growth of their children, respecting choices and evolutions in gender identity that may manifest over time.

Psychological Tools for Parents

This chapter introduces additional psychological tools for parents, providing insights on how to manage specific psychological challenges related to gender diversity. From stress management tips to the importance of emotional awareness, these tools are designed to strengthen parents' mental health.

Ongoing Family Dialogues

Gender diversity is an ever-evolving journey. This chapter explores how parents can maintain ongoing family dialogues, creating a space where open communication and mutual support are constant.

Sustainability in Acceptance

Sustainability in acceptance is a long-term goal. We explore how loving parents can maintain a sustainable commitment to acceptance, adapting to the changing needs of their children and continuing to celebrate gender diversity.

Useful Resources - Psychologists' Advice and Practical Examples

Guiding a transgender child requires constant commitment and the support of useful resources. In this chapter, we will explore psychologists' advice and provide practical examples to help parents find support and guidance.

Seeking Guidance from Expert Professionals:

Psychologists suggest seeking the support of professionals experienced in gender identity, such as psychologists or specialized therapists.

Practical Example: Scheduling regular appointments with an experienced professional can provide a safe environment to explore emotions and receive practical advice.

Participating in Support Groups:

Psychologists recommend participating in support groups to gain valuable connections with other families facing similar situations.

Practical Example: Joining online or local groups allows parents to share experiences, exchange advice, and receive mutual support.

Educating Yourself on Law and Rights:

Psychologists suggest understanding legal rights and laws that protect transgender children.

Practical Example: Organizing meetings with lawyers specializing in LGBTQ+ rights to understand the rights of the child and the family.

Building a Support Network:

Psychologists emphasize the importance of creating a support network. Friends, family, and teachers can be crucial allies.

Practical Example: Organizing educational events or sharing informative resources with the support network contributes to creating an accepting environment.

Using Online Resources and Specialized Literature:

Psychologists advise that online resources and specialized literature offer up-to-date information and success stories.

Practical Example: Creating a list of blogs, books, and documentaries addressing gender diversity enhances understanding.

Maintaining Open Communication with the School:

Psychologists recommend maintaining constant communication with the school to ensure necessary support.

Practical Example: Scheduling regular meetings with teachers and school staff to discuss the child's needs and develop inclusion strategies.

Implementing these useful resources can be a significant step in building a strong support network and addressing challenges related to the family acceptance of gender diversity. As we conclude this guide, we encourage parents to continue the dialogue, education, and promotion of acceptance within their families and the surrounding society.

In this chapter, we have examined deep family connections and the importance of sustainability in the created environment, integrating psychological tools for parents and additional educational resources. Let's now continue our journey, addressing specific challenges that may arise during the family's acceptance journey of gender diversity.

Chapter 7: Facing Challenges and Celebrating the Journey

Introduction:

In this chapter, we explore the specific challenges that may arise during the family's journey of embracing gender diversity. Addressing these challenges requires understanding, resilience, and the awareness that the journey is a continuous process of growth. Let's celebrate victories and face challenges with determination.

Tackling Common Challenges

Challenges are an inevitable aspect of any journey, and the path of gender diversity is no exception. We address common challenges that parents may encounter, such as social judgment, lack of external understanding, and cultural pressures.

Insights: Psychologists' Advice

Psychologists offer strategies to handle social judgment, including building a support network, continuous education, and practicing authenticity.

Supporting Children in Personal Challenges

Beyond external challenges, children may face personal struggles related to their gender identity. This chapter explores how parents can support their children by providing a safe haven during tough times and instilling confidence in their ability to overcome challenges.

Celebrating Victories and Progress

While addressing challenges, it is equally important to celebrate victories and progress along the way. Loving parents can reflect on their children's achievements, creating an environment where every step forward is a cause for joy and celebration.

Addressing the Role of Media and Education

The role of media and education can present unique challenges. This chapter examines how parents can critically approach how gender diversity is represented in media and education, promoting a balanced and inclusive view.

Navigating Gender Identity with Love and Understanding

In this exploration of gender identity, we've delved into crucial themes related to understanding, accepting, and supporting transgender children. With contributions from psychologists' advice and practical examples, we've aimed to provide a guide to assist parents on this significant journey.

Embracing Each Individual's Uniqueness:

The fundamental key to supporting a transgender child is to accept and celebrate their uniqueness. Psychologists emphasize that every individual is different, and unconditional acceptance contributes to the child's emotional well-being.

Creating an Environment of Acceptance:

We explored how to create an inclusive family environment, promoting diversity and open communication. The consistent practice of respectful language and active support has been identified as key tools for building a welcoming environment.

Utilizing Available Resources:

Resources, both online and local, play an essential role in providing support and guidance. Psychologists advise leveraging professional services, participating in support groups, and staying informed about legislation related to transgender rights.

Continuous Education:

Understanding and continuous education are crucial pillars on this journey. Psychologists emphasize that ongoing learning helps reduce stereotypes, promote acceptance, and foster an open mindset.

Cultivating a Support Network:

Finally, we highlighted the importance of a supportive network. Sharing experiences, participating in community events, and collaborating with schools can create an environment where the child feels supported from all angles.

In conclusion, supporting a transgender child is a deep commitment that requires love, understanding, and concrete actions. This guide aims to be a beacon of light on this journey, offering practical resources and advice to help parents create an environment where their children can fully explore and embrace their gender identity. With love, openness, and continuous commitment, we can contribute to building a more inclusive and respectful world for all.

In this chapter, we've explored the specific challenges that may arise during the family's journey of embracing gender diversity, integrating practical advice from psychologists and additional educational resources. Let's now continue our journey, exploring the diverse perspectives and voices of those who may wish to better understand gender diversity in their children.

Chapter 8: Explaining Gender Diversity to Children with Sensitivity

As we commit to supporting and understanding transgender children, it is equally important to address the questions of children who might be curious but not necessarily personally involved in gender identity. This chapter will provide tips on how to respond to children's questions about gender diversity with sensitivity and clarity.

Creating an Open Space for Conversation:

When children ask questions about gender diversity, it's important to create an open space where they feel free to express their curiosity without fear. Experts suggest responding to questions with patience and openness.

Practical Example: "I like that you're curious! Do you want to ask something about gender diversity? I'm here to answer your questions."

Using Age-Appropriate Language:

Adapting language to the child's comprehension level is crucial. Psychologists advise using simple and accessible language.

Practical Example: "Imagine that every person is like a different flower. Some flowers are big, others are small, but each is special in its own way. Similarly, there are people who feel different inside and want to be respected for who they truly are."

Promoting Acceptance and Kindness:

Encouraging children to be kind and respectful to others is a fundamental message. Experts suggest promoting acceptance of gender diversity and emphasizing that everyone has the right to be themselves.

Practical Example: "It's important to be kind to others and respect differences. People can be different, but everyone deserves respect and friendship."

Introducing Positive Stories:

Telling stories that portray transgender characters positively can help normalize gender diversity.

Practical Example: "You know, there are stories of people who feel different in their hearts, and the beautiful thing is that each of these stories is special. Can I tell you a story about how someone found the courage to be themselves?"

Addressing Specific Questions:

If the child has more specific questions about gender diversity, responding honestly and tailoring the answers to their comprehension level is important.

Practical Example: "Are you asking what it means to be transgender? It's a bit like when someone feels different from what others might think, and they want to be recognized for who they really are."

Handling children's questions about gender diversity with openness and sensitivity contributes to building a broader and respectful understanding of the world around them. Sharing these concepts in an accessible way can help cultivate an open mindset from a young age.

Final Chapter: Beyond Labels, Toward a Future of Acceptance

Introduction:

Our journey through gender diversity has been a path of discovery, learning, and, above all, love. As we close this booklet, we reflect on what we've learned and embrace the opportunity to shape a future of acceptance and understanding for all.

Final Reflections: The Uniqueness of Every Individual

Every child is a unique individual, with a unique story, path, and journey. This final chapter invites parents to reflect on the beauty of diversity and the importance of embracing the uniqueness of every individual, regardless of gender labels.

The Power of Unconditional Acceptance

We've explored how unconditional acceptance can create stronger family bonds and an environment that nurtures each child's growth. Acceptance goes beyond gender norms and social expectations, paving the way for a love that embraces individuality.

Looking Ahead: Building an Inclusive Future

This final chapter is an invitation to look ahead, to imagine and build a future where gender diversity is celebrated, understood, and respected. Change begins in families, and every small daily action contributes to shaping a more inclusive world for future generations.

A Warm Thank You

We thank you, loving parents and curious readers, for being part of this journey with us. Your dedication to love, openness, and acceptance is the foundation of a brighter and more compassionate world.

Additional Resources: Continuing the Journey

For those seeking further resources and insights into gender diversity, we invite you to check the resources listed at the end of the book. Knowledge is a powerful key to building bridges of understanding and connection.

Conclusion: A Never-Ending Journey

As we conclude this booklet, let's remember that the journey of gender diversity is never-ending. Every day is an opportunity to learn, grow, and love even more. With open hearts and curious minds, let's face the future with confidence and hope, shaping a world where every child can flourish, regardless of who they are or choose to become.

Thank you for sharing this journey with us. Together, we can build a world where every individual is free to be authentically themselves.

Additional Chapter Bonus: Exploring One's Gender and Sexual Identity

Introduction:

In this chapter, we will provide resources and advice for both adults and children who are exploring their gender and sexual identity. We'll address common concerns and provide practical tools to assist in the process of self-discovery.

For Adults:

Chapter: Exploring One's Gender and Sexual Identity

Introduction:

In this chapter, we will delve into the delicate process of exploring one's gender and sexual identity. With the guidance of a psychology professional, we will explore the need for self-awareness, reflection, and how to embark on this personal journey with awareness and self-respect.

1) Self-Awareness and Reflection:

Self-awareness is the first crucial step in the journey of exploring gender and sexual identity. It involves the awareness and deep understanding of oneself, going beyond social labels and gender stereotypes. A mindful approach involves:

- Exploring Emotions: Identifying and understanding emotions related to gender and sexual identity. What does it feel like when reflecting on these aspects of oneself?

- Reflection on Past Experiences: Analyzing past experiences related to gender and sexual identity. Which moments have had an impact on your perception of yourself?

- Evaluation of External Expectations: Examining external and social expectations regarding gender identity. How do these expectations influence your self-concept?

2) How to Start Exploring One's Identity:

Starting to explore one's identity requires a gradual and respectful approach towards oneself. The following steps are helpful:

- Reading and Information: Begin with reading informative resources on the diversity of gender and sexual identities. Books, articles, and online resources can provide a foundational understanding.

- Open Conversations: Find safe spaces to openly converse with trusted friends, family, or a professional. Sharing thoughts and doubts can be liberating.

- Participation in Communities: Join online or local communities that support the exploration of gender and sexual identity. Listening to others' experiences can be instructive.

3) Personal Reflections and Self-Awareness:

Personal reflection is a crucial aspect of the journey. Some tips to encourage it are:

- Reflection Journal: Keep a personal journal to express thoughts, emotions, and daily reflections on gender identity. This can serve as a safe space to explore oneself.

- Guided Questions: Turn to guided questions that stimulate deep reflection. What does authenticity mean to you? How do you see your identity in relation to others?

- Creative Exploration: Utilize creative forms of expression such as art, writing, or music to explore your identity. Artistic expression can reveal profound and intuitive aspects of oneself.

Conclusions:

Awareness and exploration of one's identity take time, patience, and kindness towards oneself. Through self-awareness and reflection, the door opens to a more authentic understanding of oneself, creating space for a life lived in harmony with one's gender and sexual identity.

4) Psychological Resources:

Specialized psychological counseling can be a valuable resource in the journey of exploring gender and sexual identity. A qualified professional can offer:

- Specialized Advice: Psychologists specializing in gender and sexual identity can provide targeted and personalized advice. This includes exploring emotions, analyzing past experiences, and supporting in navigating specific challenges related to identity.

- Emotional Support: Dealing with doubts and uncertainties often requires dedicated emotional support. Professionals can create a safe space to freely express thoughts, fears, and desires.

- Practical Tools: Psychologists can provide practical tools to address specific situations. This may include strategies to manage stress, improve communication with others, and promote positive mental health.

- Self-Discovery Path: Through counseling, a more structured path of self-discovery can be initiated. This involves delving into the roots of one's emotions and building a deeper understanding of oneself.

5) Professional Support for Addressing Doubts and Uncertainties:

Addressing doubts and uncertainties about gender and sexual identity can be complex and emotionally intense. Professional support offers:

- Non-Judgmental Environment: Counseling provides a non-judgmental environment to explore doubts and uncertainties without fear of condemnation. This environment facilitates open and honest communication.

- Stress Management: Dealing with doubts about identity can generate stress and anxiety. Professionals can teach stress management techniques to facilitate a smoother navigation of the path.

- Individual Action Plan: In collaboration with the client, professionals can develop an individual action plan. This may include specific steps to further explore gender and sexual identity in a sustainable way.

- Extended Resources: Professionals often have access to extensive support networks, including other specialists and organizations. These resources can be helpful in addressing specific aspects of gender and sexual identity.

Conclusions:

Specialized psychological support plays an essential role in helping individuals explore their gender and sexual identity. With targeted advice and a supportive environment, counseling provides the necessary resources to address doubts and uncertainties constructively, promoting an authentic and respectful journey of self-discovery.

6) Communities and Support Groups:

Joining online communities or local support groups is a significant step in exploring gender and sexual identity. This sharing of experiences offers:

- Empathetic Sharing: Joining online communities or local groups allows sharing experiences with people who understand the challenges and joys related to gender identity.

Empathetic sharing can reduce the sense of isolation and provide emotional support.

- Informative Resources: These groups often serve as hubs for informative resources and updates on gender diversity. Members can exchange practical advice and relevant information, contributing to ongoing education.

- Meaningful Connections: Participation in communities offers the opportunity to build meaningful connections with people who have faced similar situations. These bonds can become a source of inspiration and support during the exploration journey.

7) Sharing Experiences and Connection:

- Active Listening: In these contexts, active listening is crucial. Sharing experiences requires an environment of acceptance, respect, and mutual understanding. Active listening allows creating a space where every voice is recognized and valued.

- Virtual Connectivity: Online communities offer a unique opportunity to connect with individuals from different parts of the world. This diversity of perspectives can enrich personal understanding and foster a sense of global belonging.

- Events and Meetings: Many groups organize events, meetings, or conferences where members can meet in person. These direct interactions can strengthen the bonds created online and provide tangible support.

Practical Tips:

- Respect for Differences: Within communities and support groups, it's important to practice respect for individual differences. Each journey is unique, and the diversity of experiences enriches collective understanding.

- Conscious Participation: Engaging in discussions and sharing experiences should happen consciously. Respecting others' privacy and contributing to an environment of mutual acceptance is crucial.

Conclusions:

Joining communities and support groups provides a solid social foundation for those exploring gender and sexual identity. Connecting with like-minded individuals creates a valuable support network, contributing to a sense of belonging and shared understanding.

For Children:

8) Open and Welcoming Dialogues with Children:

Creating an open family environment to discuss gender and sexual identity is essential for children's emotional well-being.

This requires:

- Free Communication: Encouraging children to freely express their thoughts and feelings about gender identity without fear of judgment. Open communication promotes mutual understanding.

- Empathetic Listening: Practicing empathetic listening is crucial. Trying to understand children's perspectives, responding with empathy and understanding, promotes constructive dialogue.

- Normalizing the Conversation: Treating gender identity as a normal and natural topic helps reduce the associated taboo. This fosters an environment where children feel free to explore and understand themselves.

9) Inclusion in Schools:

Schools can play a crucial role in creating an inclusive and welcoming environment for all students:

- Sensible Education: Introducing educational programs that teach the importance of gender and sexual diversity. This promotes

 awareness and understanding among students.

- Anti-Discrimination Policies: Implementing anti-discrimination policies that prohibit bullying or discrimination based on gender identity. This creates a safe environment where students can express themselves freely.

- Resources for Educators: Providing resources and training for educators and teachers. These professionals can be equipped with the knowledge and tools to address children's questions and concerns respectfully.

10) Active Parental Involvement:

Parental involvement is essential to support children in exploring their gender identity:

- Openness to Discussion: Creating a family space where children feel free to discuss any topic, including gender identity. Openness fosters trust and communication.

- Parental Resources: Providing informative resources and educational materials to parents. These can help parents better understand gender identity issues and offer practical advice on supporting their children.

- Active Participation: Actively participating in children's exploration journeys. Attending school events, informative sessions, and support groups can reinforce parental involvement.

Conclusions:

Creating open and inclusive environments both at home and at school is crucial to support children in exploring their gender identity. Non-judgmental dialogues, sensitive education, and active parental involvement contribute to an environment where children feel accepted and supported.

Practical Tips for All:

11) Reading and Educational Resources:

- Book Selection: Choose books that address gender and sexual identity inclusively and informatively. Age-appropriate books can be a powerful resource to initiate discussions and promote understanding.

- Tailoring to Ages: Tailor the choice of books and resources to the readers' ages. This ensures that the content is appropriate and understandable, contributing to the building of a solid knowledge foundation.

- Active Discussion: After reading, encourage open discussions about the plot and topics covered in the books. This stimulates reflection and allows readers to express their opinions.

Responsible Online Research:

- Research Guidelines: Provide clear guidelines on how to conduct responsible online research. Encourage the use of reliable and carefully verified sources to avoid spreading misinformation.

- Awareness of Stereotypes: Warn against online gender stereotypes. Promote a critical understanding of information and encourage evaluating its reliability.

- Evaluation Guide: Offer guidelines on evaluating online sources. This may include checking the source's reputation, examining references, and comparing information with multiple sources.

Consulting Competent Professionals:

- Recognizing Signs of Difficulty: Inform about signs that might indicate the need for professional counseling. These signs may include significant changes in behavior or emotional well-being.

- Role of Professionals: Explain the role of qualified professionals in providing support. They can offer specialized counseling to address significant doubts or difficulties related to gender and sexual identity.

- Finding Local Professionals: Provide resources on how to find qualified professionals in one's area. This may include access to professional directories, local organizations, or involvement with healthcare services.

Conclusions:

Conscious use of educational resources, responsible online research, and consultation with qualified professionals are essential tools to understand and navigate gender and sexual identity in an informed and respectful manner. These practical tips contribute to building a solid foundation for conscious and informed learning.

Bonus Chapter: Identity Exploration - Thought-Provoking Questions and Reflective Test

Navigating one's sexual orientation is a personal and evolving journey. To assist children and teenagers in better understanding themselves, we present a series of stimulating questions and an optional test. These tools are designed to foster open dialogue, personal reflection, and respect for the uniqueness of each individual path.

Thought-Provoking Questions:

1. When envisioning a romantic relationship in the future, do you picture it with someone of the opposite gender or the same gender?

   - a) Opposite gender.

   - b) Same gender.

- c) I haven't thought about it.

2. What types of relationships do you find more intriguing or fulfilling in movies or books?

   - a) Heterosexual relationships.

   - b) Homosexual relationships.

   - c) Relationships don't interest me much in stories.

3. How comfortable do you feel discussing romantic feelings or attractions with friends or family?

   - a) Very comfortable.

   - b) Somewhat comfortable.

   - c) Not comfortable at all.

4. When daydreaming about a romantic partner, do you imagine someone of the opposite gender or the same gender?

- a) Opposite gender.

- b) Same gender.

- c) I don't daydream about romantic partners.

5. How do you feel about affectionate gestures like hugs or holding hands with people of the opposite or same gender?

- a) Comfortable with the opposite gender.

- b) Comfortable with the same gender.

- c) Not comfortable with physical closeness.

6. When thinking about your closest friendships, are they usually with people of the opposite or same gender?

- a) Mostly with the opposite gender.

- b) Mostly with the same gender.

- c) Gender doesn't influence my friendships.

7. What qualities do you find attractive or interesting in a potential romantic partner?

- a) Qualities traditionally associated with the opposite gender.

- b) Qualities traditionally associated with the same gender.

- c) A combination of various qualities, regardless of gender norms.

8. How important is it for you to conform to traditional gender expectations in your relationship?

- a) Very important.

- b) Somewhat important.

- c) Not important at all.

9. In your social circles, do you feel there are expectations or assumptions about your romantic interests based on your gender?

- a) Yes, there are expectations.

- b) Some expectations, but not dominant.

- c) No, there aren't any expectations.

10. When discussing "crushes" or romantic interests with friends, do you find yourself more intrigued by stories involving the opposite or same gender?

- a) Opposite gender stories.

- b) Same gender stories.

- c) I don't pay much attention to those conversations.

Identity Exploration Test:

Assign a score to each answer:

- a) = 1 point

- b) = 2 points

- c) = 3 points

Total Score:

11-15 Points: Your inclinations may align more with preferences for the opposite gender.

8-10 Points: You exhibit openness to diverse romantic orientations.

4-7 Points: Your responses indicate a balanced and open perspective towards romantic interests.

1-3 Points: Your preferences are not strongly defined at this point, and that's perfectly okay.

Note: This test is a tool for self-reflection and does not precisely determine sexual orientation. Remind parents and teachers that sexual orientation can evolve over time, so it's crucial to avoid any form of manipulation.